CURE DIVERTICULITIS: THE REAL CAUSE & CURE

HOW I COMPLETELY CURED MY SEVERE DIVERTICULITIS

By

NICOLE ROBINSON

Copyright © 2017

CONTENTS

Introduction

How to use this book

What is Diverticulitis?

The real cause of diverticulitis

What the doctors will tell you

What erodes your intestine wall

Step 1: Immediate treatment

Step 2: Resting the affected region

Step 3: Good and bad foods

Step 4: Natural remedies that cured me

How and why the cure works

Colloidal silver

Foods to eat

Foods to avoid

Conclusion

Introduction

This book explains the real cause of diverticulitis, and simple steps to cure it. The doctors know only part of the story.

It explains everything you need to know, without useless information.

I had severe diverticulitis that led to hospitalization. I was treated with emergency intravenous antibiotics. Later the doctors told me I could never cure it, and just had to "manage" it.

I followed the nutritionist's advice which helped a little, but it did not cure me. I still had occasional discomfort and pain.

I didn't accept there wasn't a cure, so I did my own research. It took about a year of research and trial and error. When I found the real cause, I made some simple changes and was completely cured within 6 months. This was confirmed by a colonoscopy and the doctors believe I was just a rare case. I'll explain everything I did.

Keep in mind my condition was quite severe. The doctors said it was "incurable". They were wrong.

The body has a remarkable healing mechanism, but what makes diverticulitis particularly difficult to heal is it is basically a bunch of holes and cavities in your intestine. You can't just fill them up with putty. They aren't going away in a hurry.

But also understand your body has many physical anomalies, and it learns to cope and adapt.

One example is my mother had a serious heart defect. The surgeons didn't know about it when they gave her a triple bypass. They were perplexed to how she had survived with the defect, but it seemed the structure of muscles had somehow adapted to the anomaly.

Put into the context of diverticulitis, curing diverticulitis may not be filling the holes in your intestinal walls. You can "manage" your symptoms by eating right.

But there are also ways to re-build the intestinal wall, which is more like a cure than plan for management.

How To Use This Book

You don't need a long book full of useless information. It is concise with clear steps to take to cure your diverticulitis. It has some important background information, but core parts are:

- The real cause of diverticulitis
- Foods to eat
- Foods to avoid
- Herbs and natural medicines that cured me

What Is Diverticulitis?

Diverticulitis is an abnormality in your lower intestines. Small pockets in the intestine linings form, which hold bacteria. The bacteria causes a painful infection. In some cases it means only mild discomfort. In other cases, it can lead to severe pain and serious complications.

The Real Cause of Diverticulitis

Doctors will tell you it's caused by a bad diet and lifestyle. It's a vague explanation.

Diverticulitis is caused by a thinning of your intestine wall. Initially the thinning looks like small pockets. If this condition isn't treated early enough, deeper pockets can form and become a more serious problem. And that's when faeces and bacteria can become trapped and cause serious infection.

What the Doctors Will Tell You

Chances are you've already been diagnosed, and been given general advice to follow. You will have a list of foods to eat and avoid. But you are just "managing" the condition instead of curing it. This is the situation I was in.

One of the main things you will hear is that low-fiber diets cause diverticulitis. This is only partially true, and the relevance of fiber is not fully understood. I'll explain why fiber is relevant later in the book.

You are reading this ebook probably because you're in the same situation.

Yes the root cause is diet and lifestyle. But the damage is already done and merely eating healthier will mostly just manage your symptoms. And occasionally you may still find the pain and discomfort often returns despite you doing everything to doctors advised.

Doctors tend to read from the same book. I'm not at all discounting the importance of professional medical help because it's very important. But doctors don't know everything. Also any official research and information about cures very slowly spread. So you need to be your own doctor too.

Don't ignore what your doctors tell you. They are not always correct, but most of the time they are. Don't put all of your faith into modern medicine. But don't put all your faith into natural cures either. Take the best of both worlds. The internet is full of inaccurate information when it comes to magical cures to diseases.

What Erodes Your Intestine Wall

Two things: acid and bacteria.

If you eat the wrong foods for long enough excessive bacteria forms in your digestive system. This erodes your intestinal wall. Especially meat causes a lot of bacteria to exist in your digestive system. If you only ate vegetables, you'll find your excrement smells more tolerable than if you ate lots of meat. This is because vegetables don't generate anywhere near as much bacteria.

Also if you consume a lot of acidic foods, you will directly erode your intestinal wall.

And if you eat an imbalanced diet, even if the foods aren't initially acidic, the imbalance will still lead to intestinal wall erosion.

So there you have: it the two main causes of diverticulitis. Next I'll explain the steps to fully cure it.

Step 1: Immediate Treatment

If your condition has worsened to the point you have severe pain, go to the hospital's emergency department. Chances are you've already been diagnosed, so explain this to the doctors.

They'll probably check your blood and urine for signs of infection, then start you on a course of antibiotics. In more extreme cases, they will keep you in overnight and on intravenous antibiotics.

Bring with you whatever you need to alleviate boredom. Hospital is a very boring place.

I also suggest insisting that they do a CT scan to check for signs of inflammation. Such a scan gives then a good idea of the affected region. Most modern hospitals now have CT scanners in the emergency department, and the scans take around 60 seconds.

STEP 2: RESTING THE AFFECTED REGION

In severe cases, restrict yourself to a clear fluid diet. Don't eat solid foods because they will lead to more bacteria, and make healing more difficult.

Follow the advice of your doctor because they will give you a good understanding of how severe your condition is. You will need a colonoscopy to know the full details of your condition. It's really not as bad as it sounds so don't be nervous.

I personally could not bare the clear fluid diet. I went 3 days with nothing but fluids, until the pain was more tolerable. Then a few months later when my condition became worse again, I continued to eat solids and again the pain subsided in about 3 days. So for me, the clear fluid diet seemed unnecessary. **I just avoided consuming particular foods and it worked out fine for me.**

STEP 3: GOOD AND BAD FOODS

Gradually start eating more of the good foods, and less of the bad foods. You'll probably find the changes you need to make aren't severe, unless your diet is absolutely terrible.

My diet was never particularly bad. Sure I love pizza and some fried food, which I may have once a week. But otherwise I'd always eaten quite healthily.

Besides once having diverticulitis, I am fit and in perfect health. **What ultimately caused my problems was such a long period of missing some important elements in my diet.** Yes a large part of it was I didn't eat enough fiber, but simply eating a high fiber diet wont cure you. I tried immediately eating more fiber but it actually worsened the problem.

So why is fiber so important? Because it controls the bacteria in your intestine. And foods with fiber tend to be more alkaline (less acidic).

At the end of this book I'll list the good and bad foods for you to include in your diet.

Before continuing, I'll explain more about what ultimately caused my diverticulitis.

I ate a reasonably balanced diet, but a few parts caused a problem. For me these were:

Too much coffee (2 cups/day): Coffee is very acidic.

Too much soda (1 cup/day): Extremely acidic.

Too much meat: I wasn't eating huge portions of meat.

Too much acidic alcohol (vodka)

Not enough fiber and alkaline foods: alkaline is the opposite of acidic.

The problem for me was more a combination of factors over a long period of time. It all came back to diet, but again simply correcting your diet will not cure you. It might reduce any pain or discomfort, but it won't cure it.

To this point, if you follow the advice and eat the right foods, you will just be "managing" your symptoms. You won't be "curing" your condition yet. Next I'll explain the cure.

Step 4: The Natural Remedies That Cured Me

This is the part doctors wont normally tell you about. Some specialists on the internet will advise them (which is how I learned of them), but none of my doctors even mentioned them.

Fixing parts of my diet managed my diverticulitis for about a year. The discomfort was tolerable, although I still had days with significant pain. I was not completely free of any discomfort until I implemented the following natural remedies:

L-Glutamine: This is a white powder you can mix in any drink. Have at least 20 grams per day. Basically it acts like a band-aid your intestinal wall. **You need to take it every day for a month or more. If you constantly forget to take it, you wont benefit.** Just mix a bit in with healthy fruit juice (not apple or orange). Guava juice is best.

Probiotics: You can get these from any chemist. They are beneficial bacteria for your digestive system. Stick with the recommended maximum dose.

Bicarbonate Soda: Get this from any grocery store. Make sure it is made for human consumption and without any aluminum. Stir half a teaspoon of it in water and drink. It is basically highly alkaline and helps neutralize excessive acid in your digestive system. But keep in mind acids are important for digesting food, so don't have too much bicarbonate soda, and don't have it within an hour of eating a meal. **If you have a particularly acidic meal or drink, then mix in a small bit of bicarbonate soda to reduce the acidity.** This doesn't give you the green light to consume anything, but it will at least help.

Dark chocolate: Full of antioxidants and helps your immune system fight infection. Just have one row of a block per day.

Aloe juice: It's not particularly cheap, but take the recommended dose daily to help sooth affected regions.

Digestive enzymes: These improve the overall health of your digestive system. Get them from any chemist.

Drink plenty of water: Have at least 1.5 liters per day (around 0.4 gallons).

The above parts in combination with a more balanced diet, and avoiding the bad foods, and some time, was all I needed to be cured.

The colonoscopy I had later was unnecessary because I didn't have symptoms, but I wanted to see if my efforts made any physical and long-lasting difference. The doctors noted that the small pockets had remarkably healed over, although there were signs of scarring. Basically the lining had been restored.

If my condition had worsened to the point where closed pockets of excrement had been trapped, then it would have been a much more serious situation. Luckily for me, the pockets were still open. And more remarkably they had shrunken significantly. So it appears clear the intestine does have the ability to correct itself to some degree, without surgery.

How And Why The Cure Works

Basically the more balanced diet prevents further damage. The glutamine acts like a band-aid for your thinned intestinal walls. The probiotics helps balance the bacteria. The other components aid the entire healing process. Your body does the rest.

It may not cure severe cases where only surgery will fix the problem.

Remember to stick with the plan. If I had severe diverticulitis and it worked for me, then it will likely work for you too.

Before you judge my approach and this book, first take my advice and see how it works out for you. Be honest to yourself about whether or not you are following the plan.

Colloidal Silver

Colloidal silver is useful in treating some conditions, and in some cases of diverticulitis it may help to fight infections. But use it very carefully because in addition to killing some of the bad bacteria, it will also kill some of your good bacteria too. There are a lot of other things to be careful of when using colloidal silver. For example, using too much of it can actually make your skin slightly grey.

I found it did help control my infection, but it is expensive unless you purchase a colloidal silver generator. Then it's actually quite cheap to produce yourself.

FOODS TO EAT

- **Bread**: Avoid white bread, and give preferences to wholemeal and bread with mixed grain. White bread has refined ingredients that are acidic and cause an inbalance of intestinal bacteria.

- **Meats**: Fish and lean meats such as pork and chicken are better options than red meat. Red meat is still ok, but remember they'll contribute to bad bacteria.

- **Vegetables**: Especially green leavy vegetables are best.

- **Fruits**: Fresh apples and pears are overall best. Avoid fruits that are high in sugar content (like oranges).

- **Yoghurt**: Low fat and organic yogurt, without artificial sweeteners helps maintain a healthy digestive system.

- **Omega-3**: Eggs and fish (Tuna and Salmon) are some of the best sources.

- **Olive oil**: mixes well with simple salad

FOODS TO AVOID

- Red meats (don't over-do it)

- Spicy foods

- Fried foods

- Processed foods (virtually all canned foods, as they have many unhealthy additives)

- Potato chips and similar snack food

- Soda drinks

- Sugar. It's in so many different foods so it's hard to avoid. Actually read the labels of food so you know.

- Highly acidic fruit juice (lemon juice)

- Foods that make you "gassy"

- Artificial sweeteners: many foods labeled "light" or "low fat" use acidic artificial sweeteners

- Coffee

Assessing Your Situation

Don't expect your condition to be the same as everyone else's. It is very important for you to have a camera up your backside so the doctors can physically see what is happening.

In most cases, it will be a non-complicated case. For example, you may have some pitting and general inflammation. If you take care of yourself, you'll probably never have the problem or pain again.

But if you have complications, such as excrement trapped in a pocket, it can cause you a lot of grief. While it may be physically flushed out, the same problem may happen 24hrs later. And if your body keeps having to deal with rotting excrement it can't get rid of, you're going to feel unwell.

It sounds nasty, and it is. So you'll need to properly assess what your problem is.

Conclusion

Depending on the severity of your diverticulitis, you may need only small changes to your diet. The more severe your case, the more ou'll need to do. Only in the most extreme cases require surgery. Your doctor and a colonoscopy will give tyou an idea of how severe your case is.

If you only had pockets in your intestine, and they aren't closed over, then you should be able to achieve the same results I did.

The advice I've given should work the same for you as it did for me, but be honest with yourself. If you don't follow the plan, don't expect good results.

Remember that your condition occurred probably because of decades of abuse to your body. For me, it took about 6 months before I was virtually completely healed with no further episodes. Now I can have any foods or drinks without any pain, as long as I don't over-do it.

Please don't judge my advice or this book until you've tried everything for yourself, and stick to the plan. And if you get the same results, I'd love to hear about it and would appreciate if you could add a review on Amazon.

On a general note about health, never rely on just Google research, or any ebook, any natural remedy, or only modern medicine. Each have a bit to offer. If you rely only on modern medicine and drugs, you'll probably only be addressing the symptoms. If you are looking at natural remedies, they may be completely useless and based on opinions of sellers. Certainly there are lots of snake oil salesman. Just remember than anyone can make a convincing website, but it doesn't mean what they're selling is any use.

If you have a final website offering some fantastic new cure, take the time to review websites that have conducted controlled studies of the claims. You may find the claims are completely bogus, or that the claims of the sellers are greatly exaggerated. In any case, don't believe everything you read, and don't pin your hopes to just one thing.

Made in the USA
Monee, IL
11 January 2024